How To Declutter Your Life And Clear Your Mind Today

Jennifer N. Smith

Table of Contents

Jennifer N. Smith

Introduction

Surely, this isn't the first book on decluttering that you have come across! You might have already read hundreds of other articles, blogs and books on this topic before stumbling over to my book – for all that I know. There might not be anything new in my book that you haven't already come across before!

So, what can I offer you that's different than the other content available everywhere?

My book isn't going to just give you tips on decluttering your life; I'm not just going to stop at "Do this" and "Don't do that". Instead, I'm going to talk about my decluttering journey with all of you. I'm pretty sure that if you are reading this book, you need to declutter some parts of your lives.

I've had a lot of trouble with buying and hoarding my whole life, and I almost never threw anything away. I am big on collecting. Over the years, I have started a number of collections instead of just focusing on one or two. I collected books, DVDs, souvenirs, posters, bookmarks, notebooks, marker pens, stickers – the list is simply endless. Once, I became interested in baking and bought more cake tins and muffin trays than I'd ever need! This went on and on with every single hobby I developed over the years: quilting, sewing, scrapbooking, crocheting, screen printing, and more. You name it, I had tried it! My collections and supplies kept on increasing and filling up my home; add to that my clothes, shoes and other belongings, and what do you get? Total chaos!

It was hard for me to properly walk inside my house, let

alone function and be productive.

I lived this way for a long time before I finally thought of decluttering, and the journey wasn't a very easy one. This book is about that particular journey I made to declutter my life, and in the process, my mind.

So go on and start this book if you are in a similar situation. If my journey to decluttering my life can inspire or help anyone else with the same problem, it would make me happier beyond belief.

Good luck!

Chapter 1: Why Declutter?

This chapter is for the people who are having second thoughts about the whole thing!

Why did I think of decluttering? Well, my entire house was full of such an immense amount of junk that it was becoming hard for me to move around. Everywhere I looked, there were possessions I barely used, clothes I never wore anymore, food that expired a long time ago, and things I didn't even need. It wasn't just by closet, my cupboards and my storage units that were cluttered and full, but every single part of my home: the couches, the bed, the tables, the walls, the kitchen counters. I couldn't move around freely because of all my stuff! **I have everything I needed at hand, except the sense of peacefulness you really need in your home.**

It wasn't just my home that was messy and overflowing, but everything else in my life! I had more on my mind than I could handle, too many responsibilities, too much to do, too many friends for me to connect with. Everything in my home, my workplace and my life was brimming, **and I was feeling suffocated.**

That was my reason to declutter: because I wanted to breathe freely!

<u>**What's your reason?**</u>

If you are doubting your decision to declutter your life, let me tell you one thing: it is absolutely normal. Almost every single thing we have in our homes had costed us money in the past, or had some memories associated with them. It's not easy to simply let go of everything just because you don't use something, don't need them, or haven't used them for a very long time. If you are going back and forth on your decision, or if you aren't sure of decluttering your life, this chapter is for you.

Let me remind you of the different reasons you might have for trying to reduce the amount of mess in your home.

1. Space, Space, Space

I can tell you from personal experience, decluttering will free up more space than you ever knew you had. When you never throw away anything, you'll find them loitering on your cabinets and closets, bed, counters and drawers. Simply by throwing away what's unnecessary and unwanted, you'll be able to free up the space you need for actual belongings.

In most cases, your clutter can physically obstruct you from moving around the house free. I've myself bought more than one cabinet and storage unit to store all the junk I had lying around. This severely used up the floor and wall space in my home, obstructing me from walking around. Every single corner and wall I had was full to the brim with things I have accumulated over the years, and it was completely ruining my home.

Decluttering can actually give you back the space you have inside your home. When we buy our house, or find something for renting, we always pay attention to the amount of space we are getting. However, most of us end up filling up that space with too many furniture and too much clutter, which can take away the breathing space we need to relax. Clear them away and you get back the home that you started with, and enough space to not just walk, but dance in.

2. Prioritize What's Important

When you go on to declutter, you might finally understand what's important for you. This doesn't just apply to your possessions, but also to the many people and the responsibilities in your life.

When you are decluttering, i.e. when you are thinking of removing certain people, possessions and duties from your life, you will be more selective of what you keep. This will show you what you truly value in your life, because you'll want to keep them with you while disposing of everything else. In the future, this will also help you to be more careful of what you buy and bring home with you, the people you want to be with, and the activities you want to spend time on.

Even if you have never thought of it, starting a decluttering journey will make it clear that you understand the priorities of your own life.

3. Save Money

When I started decluttering my closet, I actually came across a lot of clothes I had even forgotten I had. I found completely new outfits that I hadn't worm more than once; I didn't have to go shopping for clothes for the next few months after my decluttering binge!

It was the same with my books! As an avid reader, I always bought a few books at least once every month, which weren't really inexpensive. However, when I went through my bookshelves, I found at least a dozen titles I hadn't even begun, which meant that I didn't have to buy any more for a few months.

Therefore, I am pretty sure that once you start decluttering your possessions, you'll have a similar experience. You might end up finding something you forgot you had and wanted to buy again, which has happened to me more than a few times. The less you have to buy in the future, the more money you are going to save over the next few months or years.

4. Make Money

When you start decluttering, you might come across belongings that you won't just be able to use yourself, but sell to make money. I did with the stuff I discovered in my own home!

I remember that I went through a baking phrase at one time and had bought everything I needed to make a few cakes, including a state-of-the-art stand mixer, all the cake pans I could find, and more. I lost interest in baking very quickly, but had all the tools any amateur baker would love to have in their kitchen. So, I did the best possible thing under the circumstances: I sold them all to a neighbor for half the price he would have paid at a store. So you can see, I made money back.

A lot of other people I know have also made quite a few dollars by selling off what they don't need. If you are planning a yard sale, decluttering your home can be the perfect way to come up with an inventory. There should be so many things around the house that you can sell off to someone who's interested: books, DVD boxed sets, paintings you have no place on your walls for, fancy dinner plates you don't use, storage units and cabinets you don't need anymore, even old clothes you don't wear.

5. Redecorate

When there's too much clutter in your rooms, it's highly unlikely that you are paying attention to your décor. People end up hoarding or cluttering either because they think they're going to need everything one day, or because they can't stop buying what they don't even need. Either ways, you are paying too much attention to storing and buying, and not enough on decorating.

After you get rid of most of your clutter, you can finally select a decorating style. "Less is more" these days, and you can decorate your rooms better with only a few objects than with hundreds. Instead of stuffing your walls with everything, choose only a few that suits your personality and your décor style. Moving all the extra furniture, all the collections you've accumulated over the years, all the junk you never seem to let go off – it can all be a huge decoration opportunity.

6. Easy to Clean

Removing junk will make it easier for you to clean everywhere. Just imagine cleaning your dining table when you don't have thousands of canned foods and cookie jars on it; it will take mere seconds to wipe it when you don't have to pick up individual items to clean underneath them.

In the same way, cleaning, vacuuming and wiping will become easy everywhere when you don't have to deal with a lot of possessions. Cleaning your kitchen will become easier without having unnecessary pots and pans to deal with; organizing your closet will take less time if you only have clothes you wear regularly. Your bookshelf will always be dust-free if you only enough books that you have enough space for; your walls will look cleaner when there aren't dozens of photo frames hanging from them.

7. Mental Freedom

Now this is something I've experienced personally: the more belongings you have, the more emotionally tied you are to them. Even if they aren't something you use regularly – or even use at all – they'll be always on your mind. When you own too much, they become your responsibility, just like the people in your life.

Take your gadgets for example; the more gadgets you own, the more you'll be worried about not losing them. Keeping track of all the gadgets that the ordinary man owns is a hassle for everyone, something that can be easily avoided if we can only be satisfied with one or two devices. It's the same with everything else! The more we own, the more they hold us back. Letting go of everything that we don't need in our lives can be the perfect way to find some peace and freedom.

8. Make Moving Easy

To be extremely practical, the less things you own, the easier it will be for you to move. Whether you are changing apartments, city or even moving to a new country, it's easy if you don't have a lot of personal belongings. If you are relocating – across the city or to another state – simply relocating your belongings could take a lot of expense, especially if you own too many things.

On the other hand, the less amount of possessions you have in your home, the fewer hassles you have to face when moving. It might not even take you more than one trip or more than one truck to move your entire life around with you, saving you a lot of time and energy.

There you have it: all the reasons for you to start decluttering. Today. Some of them were actually reasons behind my journey to remove the unnecessary clutter in my life, and some more points. Do you need any more encouragement or are these enough for you?

They are?

Good. You can now proceed to the next chapter, where I have discussed some of the most common decluttering techniques that are both popular and effective.

Chapter 2: Popular Decluttering Techniques

The "Minimalism" Approach, and the "Four Box" Method – I'm pretty sure you've at least heard about these techniques, if not implemented them in your life. In this chapter, I am going to discuss these popular methods of decluttering, as one of them might just be the perfect one for you.

The "Minimalism" Approach

Minimalists, or people who believe in minimalism, prefer their life to be about meaningful experiences and memories instead of meaningless possessions.

Minimalism is much more than just decluttering all the useless junk in your home and getting rid of them every now and then. Minimalism is actually a method of identifying everything that's important in your life and eliminating the rest. Completely unlike the modern lifestyle that we are used to, a minimalist believes that **"less is more"**.

A minimalist only has the exact amount of belongings that they need in their lives, and nothing more. They usually don't own more than a few pieces of basic clothing, footwear, gadgets or books, cooking utensils and supplies, entertainment options or even responsibilities. Of course, the concept of minimalism has been in practice for centuries, especially among the Buddhist monks who never had more than a handful of personal possessions their entire life.

Minimalism means to live with less than a total of 100

belongings. The less a person owns, the less they have to worry about everything. Only a few possessions mean that a person can live in a smaller home and pay less rent, and not spending on unnecessary objects means that they don't have to worry about their finances. Minimalists don't believe in filling up their lives with possessions just because other people have them or because they are symbols of status; they only buy what they need.

The main object of minimalism is to focus more on experiences and living your life than to accumulate possessions. When a person isn't too worried about earning money to compete with others, they can finally be happier and less stressed in their life.

The "Four Box" Method

This method of decluttering is rightly named as it uses four boxes – four boxes precisely – to sort out everything you need decluttering; this method lets you methodically sort out everything you own into four similar boxes. The boxes are labelled "Keep", "I am NOT Sure", "Trash" and "Donate/Sell/Gift". Everything a person owns or can be found inside their home can actually be sorted into these four boxes.

The plan is to go through the different rooms of your home and sort your possessions into these boxes. The boxes should be all of the same sizes, and you need to try and fill them up equally. This means that you cannot put everything in the "Keep" box and ignore the other boxes. All the boxes need to be paid equal amount of attention as you are trying to declutter your life.

So, when you clean up your closet, try to be fair to fit all your clothes, shoes, bags and accessories into the four boxes. Keep the items that you use regularly, expensive, has sentimental value or for special occasions. Everything else can go into the "Trash", "Not Sure" and "Sell/Donate/Gift" boxes; there's a strong possibility that you will end up with a lot of items that might bring you money or help someone better than sitting in your closet.

The method should be repeated with every other parts of your home: the kitchen, the pantry, your books and documents, your medicine cabinet, your music or DVD collection, your home gym, your garage and your home office. Pretty sure you can get rid of everything that you don't need in your life, by giving them away, selling them, or giving them to your friends who might find some use for them. The "NOT Sure" boxes should be tackled when you are done with the rest of your home, and still have space for some more possessions.

Chapter 3: Decluttering your Life and Clearing your mind

Now, we've come to the main part of the book. Within this chapter, I am going to share stories and tips from my own decluttering journey, from the beginning to the end.

I have divided this chapter into multiple sub-chapters, each one dealing with different steps or phases of my decluttering journey. This was the sequence I maintained personally, but it's not obligatory. In the sub-chapters below, I have combined my own ideas with the experiences of other people who are either organizational experts or had also gone through decluttering of their own.

You can follow these exact steps, or you can simply read the book and make up your own steps. Think of my book as just an introduction to the art of decluttering, not an exact guideline. **The field is entirely yours and you get to make up the rules!**

Step 1: Decluttering your Mind

What's the most cluttered part of your life? It's not your pantry or your kitchen, or even your closet that you should worry about first. It's our mind.

Our mind is where we store the most stuff – necessary and unnecessary, both. It needs a thorough tidying up and possibly emptying just like we'd do with our closets and kitchen cabinets. However, it is not easy to do so. In fact, clearing and decluttering my mind was one of the hardest things I had to do, much harder than clearing out my entire house.

What happens when our mind is cluttered and full? We keep on obsessing over the smallest things that have no positive influence over our lives, and ignore everything that's good and happy. A cluttered mind is often restless and stressed; we become unfocused and unproductive when our minds are full. Different people are worried about different reasons: financial worries, relationship problems, professional dilemmas, health issues, mental disorders, and many more.

As a modern human being, it's almost impossible to live a worry-free life with an empty mind. From the moment that we wake up, thousands of thoughts find its way into our head, and we need to learn how to declutter them.

There's no specific way for a person to declutter their mind; the process depends on the individual who wants to clear their mind. However, I can give you some tips about the procedure, and hopefully some or all of them could be useful to you.

1. Setting up Priorities

This is something I have learned the hard way, and the long way!

We might have too many tasks, chores and responsibilities on our shoulders, but they wouldn't all be equally important. What we need to do every day is to select the ones that are most important for that day, and focus only on them. Instead of thinking about something you have to do the next week, only spend your brain cells for what's immediate and important.

To be able to prioritize your life means to be able to take back control of it. Instead of giving in to the hundreds of thoughts that pass through your head at every second, you should only focus on the thoughts that are relevant for you. This is the only way that you can keep a track on your own thoughts and not waste your entire day thinking about what's not an emergency.

2. Write Everything Down

When you start writing everything down, the pressure to remember is lessened. Anything that you have to remember later: grocery lists, birthdays and anniversaries, holiday plans, important phone numbers, meetings and playdates, ideas and future plans. You can write them down on a notebook or your phone, whichever is more convenient for you. With a mobile phone, you can set up alarms for the different appointments and meetings that you have throughout the day, so that you won't have to obsess about forgetting about them.

The average person usually stresses about the simple things in life: whether they'll remember to buy coffee at the grocery store, whether they'll be able to reach a meeting on time, or whether they'll be able to remember a certain information later. All these clutter on your mind can be easily remedied if you write them down; keep them documented and close, and you won't have to clutter your mind with them.

3. Learn to Let Go

We can't achieve everything we've planned; it's just not humanely possible. However, we can let go of our misfired plans, our regrets and our failures. In fact, a lot of what's on our mind consists of all the "only if's" and "wonder how's" that are neither very soothing nor very productive.

The relationships that turned toxic – learn to let them go; the presentations you messed up – try to forget about them; the promotion that someone else got – think about something else. If you want to have a clearer mind, it is extremely important that you let go of all the negative thoughts in your mind. It is the adverse emotions and unnecessary feelings that brings a person down. The quicker you learn to "let bygones be bygones", the quicker you can feel free.

4. Stop Multitasking

Multitasking is a bad habit most of us have! We might think we are getting a lot of work done this way, but in truth, multitasking is the opposite of being productive. Trying to concentrate on too much at the same time can mean that nothing gets done perfectly and that the same tasks takes more time; we can't really focus on anything when we are trying to do everything together.

Instead, it is much better if you try and focus on each job separately. The more you try to do, the more thoughts will cram into your head. The result? You'll not be able to do anything right. When you are working from home and watching TV at the same time, you'll also be thinking about the plot of the movie you are watching, the last movie you saw of the same actor, the other movies of this series, the location the movie was shot on, if you'd ever be able to go there on a vacation, and so on. Your entire head will be filled with thoughts and information that has nothing to do with your work, and you won't be able to concentrate on anything.

5. Take Instant Decisions

Some people I know have a really hard time making decisions; I myself had this problem. Never mind the big decisions, I needed at least 15 minutes to order coffee for myself. When making any kind of decisions, a thousand thoughts came into my mind, making it almost impossible to choose.

This was one of the first changes I made about myself when I wanted to clear my mind. Whenever the time came for a verdict, I tried to be decisive and quick, and not worry too much about the consequences. I learned to ignore all the "what if's" in my head when I made a decision, and also tried not to take too much time. It took me a while but I finally learned to be confident in my decisions, and if they were the wrong ones, I learned to live with them.

So, try and be decisive at almost every aspect of your life. Of course, some decisions in your life will require patience and contemplation, and you should take your time with them. However, there are times when you need to be quick and conclusive; otherwise, the voices in your head won't let you concentrate on anything else.

6. Learn to Eliminate

Not everything that's in your mind is equally important; you can simply forget some of them and your life will go on the same. Eliminate everything that's neither necessary nor crucial, and your mind won't be as cluttered.

The process of decluttering is based on removing everything unnecessary from your life, which also includes things on your mind. Anything that's not your responsibility shouldn't be taking space inside your mind; just learn to stop thinking about them. You might be a proactive worker, but don't waste your energy thinking about your colleague's job responsibilities. Stop listening to gossip and thinking about what's happening to other people's lives unless it is relevant to yours. Stop interfering into other's lives, even when they are your loved ones. Instead of cramming in too much information, focus on yourself and your life, and eliminate everything that's unnecessary.

A clear mind is what you need, first and foremost, to start decluttering your life. Without a fresh mind, there's no use trying to get rid of junk in your drawers and cabinets; your journey of decluttering, therefore, should start here: with a clean and stress-free mind.

Step 2: Decluttering your Workplace

Where's the one place we spend most of our time outside of the house? Our workplace, of course! Whether you work in the corporate world, own a business or work from home – your place of work needs to be absolutely perfect.

This doesn't mean that you need to fill your office up with the most expensive furniture you can find; it certainly doesn't mean you have to own more gadgets that you need or use. You don't even need to have the largest room in your office for your workplace to be flawless. To be productive, you need a place to work that will be relaxing and convenient.

Your workstation should be a place where you feel most relaxed at, which is not possible if you keep it cluttered. Ideally, there shouldn't be more than two or three objects on your table; that might not be practical but the less you have on your desk, the more you will be able to concentrate on your work. Everything else needs to be out of sight, not cluttered on your desk. If you can keep your desk organized, it won't matter if you have a massive desk or a miniature one.

Here are some steps I followed when I decluttered my desk.

1. I changed my table. If that's an option, I suggest you do the same. Instead of a fancy table, I got one that has lots of tiny drawers, big enough for a few sheets of paper. Everything I had sitting on my desk went inside the drawers. I labelled the drawers so that I'll know where everything is and don't have to rummage through every one of them. Pens, markers, staplers, paper – everything had their own place. Whenever I needed something, I knew exactly where to look!

2. I only put what's absolutely necessary on my desk – my laptop, a notepad, a small potted plant and a desk calendar. Everything

else went inside the drawers and my desk top, which was not a very big one to start with, stayed absolutely clean all day long.

3. I removed the clutter of paperwork and documents from my desk, and digitalized everything. Even the paperwork I needed a physical version of – I kept in one of my drawers or in a separate chest of drawers away from my desk. This way, I don't have to rummage through all my files and paperwork when I need something; they are all labelled and stored in my computer.

4. I used to have dozens of photographs and personal memorabilia on my desk, which was a big source of clutter. Now I have one family photograph, my favorite one, instead of a dozen. Removing my personal artifacts from my desk has really helped the clutter.

5. If you are working from home or if you have a room for yourself, do what I did and get rid of everything unnecessary. It doesn't matter how big the room is, you should have as few items in it as possible. This includes furniture, decorative pieces, photographs and posters, plants and everything else. Let the walls be empty, and let there be enough floor space without filling it up with furniture. It's better to have a sparsely decorated room than a crowded one.

6. I stopped eating at my desk, as it always made more mess than I could handle. Even on the days that I bought a packed lunch with me, I ate it someplace other than at my desk. Having lunch at my desk meant bringing in plates and water bottles, spoons and forks, drinks and ketchup; sometimes, I would forget to remove them and the ketchup bottles or the packet of chili flakes would stay on my desk for weeks. I eliminated all that simply by refusing to eat at my desk.

7. I became conscious about every single item I took out of my drawers and put on my desk, from a pen to a piece of paper. Whatever I had taken out, I remembered to put back at the end of the day, which meant my desk was always tidy when I left my workplace.

An uncluttered workplace can make a world of difference to your productivity. The more comfortable you are in your workstation, the better your performance is going to be, **as opposed as to an environment you feel suffocated in.** Decluttering your workplace should be one of the top priority in your list.

Step 3: Decluttering your Bedroom

You may not spend a lot of time in your bedroom, but it needs to be a place where you feel your most comfortable in. You can't feel relaxed in a room where you feel suffocated due to the clutter made by your personal artifacts. Your bedroom, above all the other rooms in your home, should be kept as clean and tidy as possible.

Most people have a habit of dumping everything in their bedroom: their shopping, both clean and dirty laundry, food, work documents, and much more. If you, like me, have the habit of heading straight into the bedroom when returning home, your bedroom would also be cluttered and full of unnecessary objects.

Your bedroom should only for sleeping, resting, relaxing and being intimate with your partner, and nothing else. It should be the most relaxing space in your entire house, only to be used when you need your bed. Watching television in bed, working in your bed, eating in the bedroom, using a gadget – these activities should be avoided as much as possible. If you have the habit of working or using complicated gadgets in your bed, you won't be able to relax in it much.

Decluttering your bedroom will require you to go through certain steps, just like I went through when I tidied up mine.

1. If possible, invest in a closet that has drawers and cabinets instead of open shelves and hangers. Every bit of clothes and accessories that you have should fit in nicely inside your closet, and not hanging from rods, on chairs or on your bed. Whether you have a

small closet or a large one, it should be able to completely hide your clothes and other belongings inside.

2. If you don't have a built-in closet in your bedroom, try to bring in a wardrobe or a chest of drawers in your bedroom. You can find them in a whole range of prices, types and materials. The most expensive ones are made from wood while the affordable ones are made of plastic or cloth. Whatever the material, they should be big enough to hold all your belongings.

3. Your bed should have as little clutter as possible. This means removing all the extra trimmings, the decorative pillows, and everything else that doesn't have a place on the bed. Your bed should, ideally, be made first thing in the morning and ready for you to sleep in at night.

4. Working in bed should be avoided as much as possible. However, if you have to use your laptop or any other gadget in bed, it should be removed from the bed before you want to sleep. The same rule applies for your smart phones, your tablets and e-readers. Nothing should be on your bed at any time of the day, apart from your pillows, comforters and blankets.

5. Get a bedside table that has drawers. This way, you can keep everything inside these drawers instead of on top of the table and create a clutter. There shouldn't

be anything on your bedside table except perhaps a lamp and a book.

6. Keep your walls uncluttered as well. Choose a wall to hang only a limited number of photos or paintings, but don't overdo it. A clear wall is much better than a cluttered one. If you don't have a lot of space in your closets or wardrobes, you can use the walls to hang your bags and coats. In that case, keep the artwork minimum. Using all the walls can make your bedroom feel suffocating and cluttered; so if you have to use one or two of your walls for practical storage options, keep the other walls empty.

7. Keeping a chair or a couch in the bedroom often leads to it filling up with dirty laundry, carelessly discarded after you come home. If this is the case, it is better to keep the chair out of your bedroom. No chair, no place to dump your clothes.

8. Keep a laundry basket in your bedroom, big enough to hold large number of clothes. Keep all your used clothes in the basket instead of tossing them around the room. Even if you do your laundry once a week, all your dirty clothes will be hidden from sight.

9. Minimize the number of surfaces in your bedroom. The fewer open shelves and surfaces you have, the fewer place you'll have for clutter. Don't bring in too many furniture in your bedroom, and keep only a few fixed items on the open shelves that you have. Anything that you use regularly and comes in various

sizes and shapes should ideally be kept inside drawers and cabinets.

10. Even in case of furniture, use your wall space instead of floor space. Opt for hanging or mounting bedside tables, nightstands, cabinets and lamps instead of standing ones. For furniture that need to be standing, i.e. the bed or a chair, pick furniture that have thin and long legs instead of solid ones. This will make your room seem more free and empty than it is.

Your bedroom should give you a peaceful and tranquil feeling when you walk into it, which is only possible when you don't have too many things cluttering it.

Step 4: Decluttering your Bathroom

Most of us have to do with a tiny bathroom in our homes, so there isn't usually any opportunity to do much with it. We'll all love a large, airy and decorated bathroom to use every day, but the reality is much different for most people.

Bathrooms can become cluttered extremely fast, mostly because we have to store a lot of supplies in a small place. Shampoos and conditioners, makeup, soaps and towels, medicines and tissues – there are a lot of things you need to cram inside a tiny bathroom, and not much space to store them.

We had two bathrooms in our house, a small one and an even smaller one. They were cramped to say the least, and we had to rummage through tons of stuff just to find something. These are the steps I took to declutter my bathrooms.

1. I emptied it. I took away every single thing that was removable from my bathroom to sort through them. Once my bathrooms were truly empty, could finally see the exact amount of space I had for my things.

2. I threw away everything that was almost empty, really old, expired, or had less than one use left. Tons of near-empty shampoo and conditioner bottles, expired or unnecessary medication, old makeups no one uses anymore – I threw them all away without a second thought. What I had left was less than half the number I started with.

3. I threw out free samples of makeup and lotion I knew no one was going to use. There were unopened items that we had gotten as gifts from friends that were almost expired and taking up unnecessary space. I threw most of them away and gave away some to people I knew would use them.

4. Beside the toothbrushes that we actually use, there were ten to twelve others that hadn't been thrown out yet. They never made it back to the bathrooms again.

5. Next, I got rid of the mirror on my bathrooms and got the ones that come with cabinets. With these cabinets, I got both a mirror and ample space behind it for all my stuff. I could keep all my bottles and jars inside and they'd be completely out of sight.

6. I used to shop for the whole month at one time, which meant multiple bottles of the same or similar product in my toilet. This took up a lot of space unnecessarily in my bathrooms and made a clutter. After decluttering, I don't make the same mistake. I keep only one quantity of everything in my bathroom and the rest go into storage.

7. I put all my spare products in baskets, and keep them hidden away from plain sight, but inside the bathroom. There are a few places you can keep these boxes – under the bathroom sink, on shelves installed over the door, ladder shelves over the toilet, or anywhere else. As long as you store them in similar

boxes, your spare products won't clutter up the bathroom.

8. Since I had two bathrooms, I divided up my products between them. I kept our personal medications in one bathroom and all the general ones in the other one; I divided the towels up into two bathrooms. The heavy makeups were kept in one bathroom, and the ones that were used every day were kept in the other bathroom. This way, everyone knew which bathroom to use on which occasion, and none of them became too cluttered.

9. A lot of different smart organizers are available for the bathroom if you just know what to look for. For our towels, I choose a vertical mounted towel holder, as opposed to hang them all. I can keep up to half a dozen towels in each of these holders easily, and taking one out is convenient.

10. Keep similar items together, in storage or inside your bathroom cabinets, and create exact locations for them. This way, you'll know, at a glance, just what you'll need to buy on your next trip to the grocery store; you can also decide on the size of the bottle or jar you can buy based on the space you have available.

With everything that we do inside, bathrooms are hard to keep tidy and organized, even more so when there is too much clutter in it. Decluttering your bathroom will help you keep it clean at all times, so that the time you spend inside the bathroom doesn't feel suffocating.

Step 5: Decluttering your Kitchen

The kitchen in the first place around the house that gets the most cluttered, most probably because we keep on buying supplies for it almost every day. Ready food, ingredients, tools and supplies, kitchen appliances and gadgets, Tupperware, plates and bowls, pots and pans, knives, spoons and spatulas – there's almost no limit to what we need to use in the kitchen. Sometimes, even the largest kitchen won't be enough to hold everything that we need to buy for our cooking and baking needs.

Decluttering your kitchen won't be an easy job. In fact, this is the room you'll need most time and energy to deal with.

Here are some tips for when you start decluttering your kitchen. I've used some of these tips myself and borrowed others.

1. Take out all your Tupperware boxes and match them with the lids. If you are anything like me, most of them wouldn't have lids; alternatively, there will be lids but no boxes. You first step should be to get rid of all these mismatched lids and boxes. I remember holding on to them for years in the hope of finding the missing pieces, but that has never happened.

   So get rid of the lids that don't have boxes, and the boxes that don't have lids. If possible, get an entirely new set of Tupperware of the same shape and size. This will save time in trying to match lids to the boxes, and will also look good in your kitchen.

2. Get matching jars for your supplies for the kitchen, large ones for grains, pasta, rice or sugar, and small ones for spices. With matching jars, you can keep them on your kitchen counter and they won't look bad. Besides, if you put everything in jars and assign a particular location for every single one, you'll know what to buy and how much to buy. Spare food packets of different shapes and sizes won't be lining your kitchen counters unnecessarily.

3. Most people use the Internet for recipes these days. If you have a few favorite recipes in the cookbook, you can simply copy them in a notebook or take a photo of it. Cookbooks have simply become an unnecessary clutter in the kitchen.

4. If you have a moderately large kitchen, you can assign different areas of the kitchen for different purposes. For example, the area beside the stove would only be for cooking, and the area beside the sink would be for cutting and washing. This way, you can keep all the spatulas and wooden spoons beside the stove and the knives beside the sink. In the same way, a separate section for the blender, mixer, coffee machine and food processor will make it easy to work, and a separate section for baking will have all your cake pans and muffin trays.

5. If possible, install drawers and cabinets under the kitchen counters, so you can hide everything behind

the doors and panels. If your kitchen counters are empty and clean, your kitchen will look less cluttered. It will also be easy to give it a good wipe every day.

6. Keep cutlery inside drawers. You can buy sorting trays with compartments or build compartments into your drawer to keep your spoons, forks and knives separate.

7. Instead of keeping all your appliances and gadgets on the counter, keep them hidden inside counters. Apart from the coffee machine, you won't need your other appliances every day. Bring them out only when you need them, and you'll be saving a lot of space on your counters.

8. Keep just as many plates, bowls, glasses and coffee mugs as there are members in your house. Keeping more will only increase the number of dirty dishes in your sink. If everyone has a specific tableware in their name, they'll be responsible to clean it themselves after every use. Keep the extra under the counters.

9. Make sure to keep at least two to three junk drawers for everything that doesn't fit in anywhere else. Emergency candles, cake knives, cupcake molds, baking sheets, extra batteries, tongs, phone chargers, napkins, charging cords – these can be found in these "junk drawers". Anything that you can't throw away but may only need occasionally can be put in these drawers.

10. Don't keep more than two dish towels hanging from the kitchen cabinets. Wash them regularly so that you can keep on reusing them. This helps to always have a clean dish towel at hand when you need one. Get rid of other dish towels, especially the ones that are old and greying.

11. Buy your mixing bowls in sets. This way, you can keep the smaller ones inside the larger ones, and store more than half a dozen bowls in the place needed to store one. If you have mixing and baking bowls in various shapes, get rid of them or give them away.

12. Minimize the kitchen appliances that you need for preparing your meals. If you have a state-of-the-art blender, you won't need a separate coffee grinder, food processor or a juicer. Your blender will come with all the attachments needed for multiple jobs. So, you can probably get rid of all the excess kitchen appliances you don't really need. In the same way, if you don't like spending a lot of time cooking and preparing your meals, you probably won't need a pasta maker or a food hydrator.

13. Modern appliances are compact, smaller and build for storing in small spaces. They are also multi-functional; this means that updating your decade-old kitchen appliances for something modern will save you space.

14. Some kitchen appliances are simply unnecessary, i.e. a banana slicer, an egg separator, an apple slicer, a pair of salad scissors, a corn silk remover, etc. These

tools don't do anything that you can't do with a good knife, so you can probably give them all away and save a lot of space.

15. Use the cabinet doors to store everything from your spatulas to can openers. Simply by adding hooks to the inside of cabinet doors, you can hang anything that's light and small from them, i.e. measuring cups, silicon spatulas, strainers, peelers and knives, beaters and mixers.

16. Some coffee mugs and tea cup sets are only kept because of their sentimental value, not because we use them. Only a few coffee mugs and cups are actually needed in a home, and the rest of them can be given away or stored somewhere else.

17. Store kitchen items you don't regularly use somewhere else, like in the attic or the basement. Fancy tableware, for example. These are only used when you have very special coming for dinner, not every day. For when you don't need them, fancy dinner plates and casserole dishes can be stored carefully in a labeled box and kept away from the kitchen.

18. With some tools, you don't need more than one. Vegetable peelers, tea strainers, egg beaters, cutting boards, bread knives, oven mittens, set of measuring cups, cleavers, ladles, mortar and pestle – you don't really need multiple pieces of these tools. If you have

more than one, you can simply get rid of the piece that is old or outdated.

19. Instead of buying pasta in three different shapes, stick to one; you can try the other shapes when you have finished the first one. In the same way, stick to a particular type of rice or flour instead of experimenting. This will help you to store your ingredients easily in jars.

20. If possible, cover your open shelves with wooden doors so that you can't see what's inside. If installing cabinet doors isn't possible, cover them up with short curtains in matching colors. This may not help with the decluttering, but it will help with keeping your clutter hidden.

There's a good reason that kitchens are the hardest to declutter; there are simply too many types of items in a kitchen to declutter them randomly. With kitchens, it is better to learn to organize what you have instead of just blindly throwing everything out. **Decluttering your kitchen can make you frustrated, but if you stick to it, a decluttered kitchen is definitely a huge achievement.**

•

Step 6: Decluttering your Fridge/Pantry

You might have a whole room to use as a pantry, or you may only have a few drawers, but most pantries tend to get cluttered sooner or later. With everything that we need to buy for our family, space can be an issue for most homes. It's the same with refrigerators; even if you have a massive fridge in the house, it can get cramped very soon.

Cooking and baking ingredients, frozen food, canned food, chocolates and chips, cookies and ready-to-eat meals – the list goes on and on when you go shopping for food. We come back with grocery bags full of food and sometimes, there's no place to keep store them all.

This is something that had happened to me dozens of times. I've gone shopping for the essentials, and come back with more food than I needed. However, that wasn't the problem; the problem was storing the food. I had a medium-sized pantry, plenty of cabinets in the kitchen and a massive kitchen, and I still had trouble storing my groceries. The problem, I realized later, were my organizational and decluttering skills.

Here's what I learned from my journey in decluttering my pantry and fridge.

Decluttering your Pantry

1. First of all, you need to completely clear out the pantry. This means taking out everything you have

stored in your pantry, or your kitchen cabinets assigned for your groceries. You need to start fresh if you want to declutter.

2. Look through everything that you already have in your pantry and sort through them. Anything that has expired or gone bad should directly go to the bin. If you are anything like me, you'll find a lot of expired cans and jars in your pantry, forgotten and unopened. Unfortunately, these should be tossed into the garbage bin immediately.

3. You might also come across a few items that are nearing the expiration date. If they still have a few weeks or months to go, you don't have to throw them away. These should ideally go into a separate pile, to be used up within the next few weeks. You can plan your next meals based around these ingredients so that they don't go to waste.

4. Next, make a list of all the ingredients that have been gathering dust on your shelves for a few months. This could be because you don't use them in your meals anymore. Make a note to never buy them again the next time you go grocery shopping.

5. Make a second list of everything that you have left in your pantry, and an approximate estimate of how many days of use you have left of them. That is, if you want to use the ingredients already in your pantry! If you don't feel comfortable using the ingredients you already have, you can give them away to someone else or throw them away. However, since I was never a fan

of wasting food, I preferred to first use what was already in my pantry.

So, make an approximate estimation of how many meals you can prepare with the ingredients, and try not to go grocery shopping for those days. However, that decision will depend on what you find in your pantry. If all that you can find was spices and canned food, you'll of course need to shop for other ingredients. What I did, though, was to plan my meals accordingly so that I could finish the ingredients in my pantry first.

6.   The next time you go shopping, try buying products from the same brand, especially canned food. Whether you are buying canned mushrooms, peaches, baby corn or beans, buying from the same brand makes it easy to stack them. All the cans from a brand are designed so that they can be stacked one on top of another, and you can simply stack them in the same way in your pantry.

7.   Store similar items together; if possible, put them inside similar jars and bottles while storing. This is especially true for cereal, flour, grains, rice, beans or nuts. If you empty the original packets and put the ingredients in similar-looking transparent jars, you'll know exactly how much you have. This will stop you from double-buying or unnecessary stocking the next time you go to the grocery store.

Decluttering your Fridge

It's the same with decluttering your fridge. Over time, you may find food in a box at the back of your fridge that you don't remember putting. This happens more in the bottom shelf of the fridge where we don't always look regularly. Besides, we have the clutter at the top of the fridge to deal with, as well as the clutter at the front.

Decluttering the inside of your fridge means to empty your fridge, and to sort through the content. There might be boxes inside that are few weeks old, forgotten ingredients and leftover food. It's better to simply throw them away, then to eat food that has been in the fridge for several days. You might see the same inside the fruits and vegetable drawer; there might be a dried tomato or a few molding berries in a corner, forgotten from months ago. These also need to be thrown away.

Another important place to check would be the spices and condiments segment of the fridge, where you might find some of the products expired or nearing expiration date. They need to be thrown out immediately; or, if they still have a few weeks to go, finished immediately.

The same can happen in the covered section of the fridge where you keep your milk, butter, cheese, yogurt and similar contents. These products don't come with a very long shelf life and they need to be checked often. Throw away the ones that seem to be going bad, has a bad smell coming from it or is nearing the expiration date. Sometimes, we end up buying too much and can't finish them on time; it is better to throw them out than to keep them rotting in your fridge.

The inside of your fridge will get cluttered more if you are not using transparent boxes. With transparent boxes, you'll know what's inside the moment that you open the door; with any other boxes, you'll have to open the lids to know, and they get overlooked most of the times. Replace all your solid boxes with transparent ones, and you'll know exactly what's inside your fridge at all time.

In the same way, a clutter on top of your fridge doesn't look very aesthetic. If you need to store something on top, get a large basket that fits everything inside.

The front of the fridge also gets cluttered if you use it to hang everything from report cards to to-do lists. For a clean and clutter-free fridge front, keep the contents minimum. Instead of displaying everything, choose one or two every week. Better yet, alter the pattern completely and only place a few fridge magnets on it.

The fridge and the pantry are the two most frequented and visited parts of the house, While the pantry may be covered and private, the fridge is present for the whole world to see. It is almost crucial that you keep them clean and organized.

Decluttering the pantry and the fridge shouldn't just be something to do once a year, but something every family should do every few days. Decluttering will save you a lot of food from going bad, as well as save a lot of money for the next few times you go grocery shopping.

Step 7: Decluttering your Closet

Cleaning out your closet may be the hardest or the easiest part of the house, based on the person that you are. If you love clothes and treasure the contents of your closet, it will be hard for you to let go of some of them.

Decluttering your closet isn't just about making space for new clothes; it is more about prioritizing and organizing a very important part of our life. Most of us have a large wardrobe but still can't find anything we want to wear. It's a paradox actually: the more clothes we have, the less we can find to wear. The problem, as it seems, isn't about having "nothing to wear", but about "having too many options".

Rummaging through your closet will tell you exactly what you have, and help you prioritize. Most of the time, we are holding on to clothes we no longer plan on wearing but that other people might find useful. By hoarding clothes, we are not just wasting space in our closet, but misusing resources.

Whatever your reason for decluttering your closet, these are the steps that can help you.

1. The first step, as always, would be to empty out your closet. This may be done in one day, or it might take several days to complete; you can empty your whole closet all at once, or tackle the different segments of it. Whichever method you choose, your closet needs to be stripped from top to bottom, everything from the winter coats to your underwear needs to be taken down.

2. First to throw away should be everything that are torn or in rags. As opposed to clothes we have never worn, there are also some clothes that we have worn so much, they are nothing more than pieces of rags. They need to go, immediately. Most of the time, they are so worn, you can't even donate them to charity.

3. Next to go would be the old clothes that no longer fit us. Still, we hang on to them in the hopes of being able to wear them again, but that doesn't usually happen to a lot of people. There's absolutely no practical reason to keep them around. If you ever reach that target body, you'll be able to alter your present-day clothes or buy new ones. You don't have to throw them away when you can donate them, as there will be other people who need your old clothes more than you.

4. If you are keeping some of your clothes for sentimental reasons, you are simply wasting space. If you want the memories, you can simply take a photograph of yourself wearing the clothes and hang on to them, giving the actual clothes to someone else who needs them. At the most, you can keep one or two of these items for sentimental value, but let go of the rest.

5. Parents sometimes keep their children's old baby clothes in their closet, but that can use up a lot of space. Baby clothes don't actually belong in your closet; they should be properly preserved in an airtight box someplace safe, i.e. in the attic or the basement.

6. If you have too many winter coats and jackets that you don't need for long stretches of time, they can also be taken out of the closet and stored somewhere else. Jackets and coats can be hung from rails in your attic, by putting them inside plastic bags or coat bags. This will free up a lot of space in your closet and you can also bring them down at any time.

7. If you have designer bags, dresses or couture pieces that doesn't fit you or that you don't wear anymore, you can always sell them. There are a lot of people online who would love to get their hands on some exclusive pieces – even second hand and old – for reasonable price. You might actually make some money off the clothes and bags gathering dust in your closet.

8. Other old pieces of clothes that you don't plan on wearing again can simply be donated to charity or thrift stores. If you are a fashion-conscious person, you might not wear the same clothes for long or wear clothes from a few years ago, but they can help other people who need clothes.

9. There are some "useful clothes" you can never have enough of, i.e. a plain white T-shirt, black leggings, the legendary little black dress, white socks, a neat black blazer. Over time, you might just end up with half a dozen of each. Too many! Just keep two of each and donate the rest.

10. Clothes that are too difficult to maintain should also make the cut. Silk shirts that need to be ironed every

time you wear them, fluffy dresses that take up a lot of space – they are simply not worth the space or the energy.

11. There could be a few clothes that are old but you are still not ready to part with them. Keep them apart. Wear them repeatedly for the next few weeks until you are sure you have exhausted their use, and then you can give them away.

12. If you have enough work clothes but still feel the need for some new ones, swap with a friend instead of going shopping. This way you are simply replacing your clothes instead of adding more; both you and your friend gets new clothes and everyone wins.

It's not going to be an easy job – to declutter your closet and let go of clothes that were important to you at some point of your life. Get a friend to help you decide, and it will be easier; besides, think of the closet space you'll be able to free and all the people you'll be helping with your clothes.

Step 8: Decluttering your Shoes

If you are truly the fashionista, this should be another challenge for you. Personally, I wasn't bothered by cleaning by shoe storage unit because I never had too many. This was an easy part of the challenge for me. However, I do know other men and women who'd probably have a breakdown if they are asked to get rid of their shoes.

Ideally, you shouldn't own more than 5 to 6 pair of shoes, one of each type or purpose. The reality is quite different, I am aware of that. Shoes are as much a fashion accessory these days as your clothes or your bag. I have friends who own more than 50 pair of shoes, men and women both! So if love your shoes, you're going to have trouble deciding on what to keep and what to discard of.

Storing shoes can always be a problem, even when you have a separate shoe storage unit. Fancy shoes are best kept inside their boxes, which means that they end up taking more space than they should. Keeping them in your closet would also be a waste of space, unless you have a massive closet space. Even so, keeping dozens of expensive shoes lying around requires a great amount of maintaining, cleaning and airing, and no one has that much time these days.

So, if you have made up your mind to declutter your shoes, these are the steps to follow.

1. First, of course, take out all your shoes – the ones that were safely and lovingly kept in boxes, as well as the

ones you wear to run, and the ones you wear while gardening or doing something equally murky. Every single pair of shoes that you own, as well as the ones owned by your family members, need to be taken out of the cupboards, under the bed, inside the closets and behind doors.

2. Sort them into types and purposes: one segment for your party shoes, one for office shoes, one for your running shoes or sneakers, and one for miscellaneous use. Or you could make sub-segments for heels and flats, based on color or shape, or any other categories. If you are sorting the shoes for the whole family, you can ask them for making segments of their own.

3. Start with the shoes that are worn out, outdated, scratched or torn. There's every chance that you are not going to wear them again soon, so there's no use keeping them in your shoe storage anymore. You can simply throw them away, or donate them. The fancy shoes can be given to thrift shops where they'll be sold for a very reasonable price to the less fortunate people.

4. Try on the shoes you have remaining. Do you like the way they look on your feet? Do you feel comfortable wearing them? Are they still fashionable? Do you have any clothes that could be worn with these pairs? If most of the answers are "no", it's time to let go of them.

5. Do you have two or more pairs of shoes that look almost the same? The classic black stilettos or the leather boots, white strappy sandals or running shoes – these are the kind of shoes we all have multiple pairs of. Keep the one that's the most comfortable and new, and discard the others.

6. Think about the last time you had worn each of them. Last month, last summer, last year? If you haven't work a pair of shoes even once for at least 12 months, you don't really need them in your life.

7. Sort by color. You don't need more than three pair of shoes in the same color. Most of the time, the shoes we see in our collection are black, white, beige or tan, as well as other colors. Depending on the type, try to sort through the shoes of the same color.

8. Give priority to the shoes that can be worn on different occasions and with different kinds of clothes. Sneakers, for example, can be worn both while running and when you are out for chores; flats can be worn both with jeans and summer dresses. Boots can be worn with skirts, dresses and jeans, and on more than one occasion. These are the kind of multifunctional footwear that you need to hold on to, and discard the ones that are not very practical.

9. If you find shoes that are relatively new and completely unharmed, but you don't know if you'll ever wear them again, you can always sell them online. There are hundreds of websites where you can advertise your shoes and sell them at half or three-

fourth the original price. Not just that, you can swap your old shoes with other people and end up with new models you haven't worn yet.

10. Put the shoes back into your storage unit, and then, if you have space available, go through the maybe pile. You can find other pairs to keep for the time being if there's space left for any.

No one needs more than half a dozen pair of shoes in their life, but we usually end up with tons more. Decluttering your shoes can be quite hectic, but when you are done, you'll be left with what's important and necessary in your life.

Step 9: Decluttering your Laptop

It's true that the content in your laptop doesn't take up any physical space, but it can make your device slow. A cluttered laptop isn't really productive, and it can make it hard to navigate; if your work is stressful, a chaotic and slow laptop will only add to the stress.

It doesn't take a long time to declutter your laptop; neither does it require any other appliances or tools. You can simply take a few hours out of a day off to declutter your laptop, and make it as fast as it was in the beginning.

Start with the Desktop. You don't need more than a few icons on your desktop for work; everything else is simply unnecessary. Only the icons you use regularly should be distributed between the desktop and the taskbar, not on your wall. Anything else you want to use can be found on the "Start Menu" in the list or pinned to the menu. All that should be visible on your desktop are less than a dozen programs that you need to use every day.

Change your Desktop Image to Something Simple. A complicated and vividly colorful photograph on the desktop will only add to the clutter. Choose something with less than five basic colors, just to be subtle.

Clear out the Browser Extensions. With all the browsers that you use, you'll get options to install dozens of extensions. You won't need most of them in your work, so there's no need to keep them installed at all times.

Settle on One or Two Browser. You don't really need more than one browser to access the Internet, so that's all you need. You can keep another one just for emergencies.

Limit your Startup Buttons and Tasks. If you have a lot of startup tasks, your laptop would automatically start them when you turn on the device. This will make the laptop slow to navigate from the very beginning. Reduce your startup tasks to only one or two; you can start the others manually when you need them.

Uninstall the Apps and Software you don't Use. No one uses all the apps they have installed on their laptop, so you can simply delete them. If you open the "Add/Remove Programs" from "Control Panel", you can see a list of everything that is installed in the computer. You can easily uninstall and delete the ones you don't need from the list.

Delete Movies. If you have movies and TV series saved in your computer that you are done watching, delete them.

Sort out the different drives. Assign each drive for different purposes. You can get more than half a dozen drives in your laptop, depending on the RAM size. Keep files and documents of different types in each drive, i.e. one for work documents, one for photographs, one for videos and one for your important documents.

Keep Photos and Videos somewhere else. If you have a lot of personal videos and photographs saved in your computer, transfer them to an External Hard Drive for safekeeping. A handful of videos can take up a large amount of space on your computer and make it slow.

Name your Folders Accordingly. If you want to find out where everything is quickly, you need to name them accordingly, preferably with dates. We may simply name a document or a folder "XYZ" or "bdyyff" when we are in a hurry, but it will be hard to locate later.

Clean your Recycle Bin. Whatever we delete from our computer stays in the Recycle Bin, and we need to clear the bin at least once or twice every week.

Use "Disk Cleanup". Using this app will delete all the temporary Internet files, cookies, search history, system error logs and other unnecessary files from your computer. This is the only way to delete these files; you cannot remove them manually.

Unsubscribe to Unwanted Emails. We all subscribe to various newsletters on different websites, but they become annoying over time. Take your time to unsubscribe to all of them, so that these undesirable emails don't take up space on your email account.

Take my word for it: you'll actually feel lighter when you've decluttered your laptop or computer from these unnecessary junks. No, it won't make the laptop physically lighter when you clean it up, but it will make working easier.

Step 10: Decluttering your Phone

Your phone works in almost the same way as your computer, especially if you are using a smart phone. Just like a laptop, your phone will also become slow and unresponsive if you fill it up with clutter and junk.

We use our smartphones more than we use any other device, which is why it tends to get overwhelmed more. A cluttered phone is a slow one, and it could seriously compromise your operating quality. Your phone may just get hung up when you are about to reply to an important email or answer an emergency call.

It is very important to keep your phone as clean as possible, which you can do by these following steps.

1. With the Play Store and the App Store full of free apps, we can find ourselves downloading a new one every day. Although they are free, all these apps take up valuable space in your phone. Deleting these unnecessary and unused apps can be a great way to clean your phone. You can install them back anytime you need to use them, if you have access to the Internet.

2. Not every single app needs to be on your phone's home screen. You can keep them hidden inside folders for when you need them. This feature is available in most phones, but if your phone doesn't have it,

you can download special apps that lets you do exactly that.

3. You can create folders based on the different types of apps, or based on their usage. Your most used apps can go in one folder, like your camera, ride sharing apps or financial management apps. Alternatively, you can arrange them based on what they are used for, i.e. one folder for apps to order food, one folder for camera and photo editing apps, one folder for Social Media and one folder for your official communications. You'll know exactly which folder to go into when you need to use your phone.

4. Smartphones are great if you like taking photographs; you'll have a good camera with you at any time of the day. However, too many pictures and videos stores in the phone will use up valuable space and make your phone slow. Every now and then, it is important that you transfer the photos and videos to your laptop, to an external hard drive, or upload them to a cloud account.

5. If you love playing games on your phone, make sure that you haven't downloaded too many of them. Some games are quite big in size; they can use up a lot of space on your phone and there are a lot of smaller games as well that doesn't need as much space, too. If you are installing the larger game

apps, it is important that you don't install more than two or three.

6. Instead of storing music on your phone, you can use an app that lets you stream your favorite songs. There are several options for you to choose from, **Spotify** is the most popular option for streaming movies. **YouTube** has all your favorite music as well.

7. It's the same with movies. In the previous decade, we used to store movies and episodes of our favorite TV series on our phones, but you can stream them from your phone these days.

8. Go through your phone book and delete the contacts you never use. The same should be done with your phone messages.

Now, your smartphone is a device that you hold in your hand every day, so it should be as productive as it can be. A cluttered phone will become slow and unresponsive, which can be annoying. Decluttering your phone isn't going to take long, either; you can even do it on the go or while watching TV.

Step 11: Decluttering your Social Media

Most people spend an insane amount of time on their social media accounts these days, checking up on their friends and family members. For some, it has become an unhealthy obsession over time; they can't seem to stay away from their social media account, no matter how much they try. Whether they are following the lives of others intensely or sharing every single aspect of their own lives, Social Media has become a fixation for some people.

Decluttering your Social Media accounts can be a good way to make sure you are spending less time on them. This is something I had struggled with personally, and these are the steps I had followed in my own life.

1. Depending on how active you are on your social media accounts, it might take you one or several mornings to declutter your digital life. It's better you start on a weekend morning when you have enough time on your hands. That's what I did.

2. I start with the social media account I use the most. Over time, we add a lot of people to our account, even though they aren't close to us. Sometimes, we even add people who aren't our direct acquaintances simply because we've interacted with them online. It is actually quite dangerous to add people you don't know, especially if you are sharing information and pictures of your family. You should start your decluttering by removing these people. It might take

up to an hour if you have a large number of friends, but it is an important step.

3. Next, you should try to remove the people you knew once personally but actually aren't in touch with, emotionally or physically. Ex-romantic partners, people you used to work with ten years ago, people you went to school with but can't even remember, neighbors you used to live beside, fourth cousin twice removed – these people don't have to be in your friend-list. People you knew at least 20 years ago but no idea about at the present shouldn't be privy to your personal information.

4. If you regularly share pictures and information about your family, especially your children, some people shouldn't be on your list. These are people you don't really trust or feel comfortable about.

5. Go through all the pages, celebrities and media personalities that you follow. If there are some you don't really like or agree with at the moment, unfollow them.

6. If there are people in your friend-list who always post negative, hurtful, biased, racist or sexist content, it will be better to "Unfriend" or "Unfollow" them; you can also choose not to see any post from them.

7. If you are a member of groups that aren't relevant to you or that you aren't interested in anymore, take leave from those groups.

8. If you have more time on your hands, go through all the contents you had posted during your early years. You might want to delete some of your posts that you would be embarrassed about now. You can also go through the photos you have posted or that other people have tagged you in, and filter them.

You can use the same steps in decluttering your social media account we share our personal life on, and I guarantee, you'll feel much lighter after you are done.

Step 12: Decluttering your Walls

Yes, that's right! Your walls can get cluttered too if you put too much on them. Too many photographs on your walls, too many posters or paintings, too much color, too many vacation memorabilia or souvenirs – these can all make your walls look cluttered. Decorating doesn't always mean putting everything you have on display; most of the time, subtlety is better. Especially in case of your walls, the less you put on, the better your walls look.

Here's how you declutter your walls:

1. Focus on one particular wall of each room. Use that one particular wall to put on your paintings, photographs and other decorative pieces instead of using all four walls. You can use the other walls for different uses, but don't make collages of photographs and paintings in multiple walls of the same room. If more than one wall of a room has a collage on it, completely empty them except one.

2. Floating shelves on your wall are a better option than buying cabinets or bookshelves. These shelves don't crowd your rooms and gives you the perfect opportunity to display your books and souvenirs. It is better to install a few floating shelves on your walls than buying more furniture at triple the price. However, it is also important not to overdo it. Two to three floating shelves on a single wall is better than

installing half a dozen simply because you have the space.

3. Open shelves, book shelves and floating shelves are for display only, not for storage. Everything that you keep on these shelves should be arranged in an aesthetic manner. One of the biggest mistake everyone makes is to overcrowd these open shelves with too many objects, which can clutter up a room. Each shelf shouldn't have more than two to three objects on display, depending on the length of the shelf, or more than a dozen books.

    The more you display on your open shelves, the more cluttered your walls are going to feel. So if you have more than the required number of objects or books on display, remove them. You can alternate between your favorite pieces every week, but don't place them together.

4. If you want to paint your walls a darker shade or if you want to apply decorative wallpaper on your walls, don't do it on more than one or two walls in each room. At least majority of the walls should be painted in a lighter shade if you want to paint the fourth one dark, or apply a vivid wallpaper to it.

5. If your collage of photographs or paintings on one wall is looking cluttered, changing the frames might help. Change the decorative and thick frames to something simple and slim, and your walls would look less cluttered.

6. Instead of half a dozen paintings on a wall, choose one. It can be a large one in the center of the wall, highlighted by spotlights.

7. Not every single wall needs to be decorated, painted in vivid colors or adorned. Some of them can simply be left alone with nothing on them. In fact, it helps to make your room less cluttered.

8. Experimenting with lights can actually be considered a kind of art. Some of your walls can simply have a light or a lamp hanging from it to decorate it, and nothing else. There's a different kind of beauty in empty, unadorned walls.

9. If you have large windows filling up your whole wall, it's completely okay to keep it natural. Change your curtains to light fabric in subtle colors to keep the view natural, and the room will feel less cluttered.

10. If something on your walls doesn't feel right or demands your focus every time you look at it, remove it.

What you do with the walls in your home depends completely on your personality and preference. If you want to keep them completely empty, that's also up to you. In fact, walls shouldn't be crowded and cluttered. Your walls shouldn't make you feel suffocated; they should be peaceful to look at. If something doesn't feel comfortable, take it out. Decluttering your walls should be something that comes to you naturally.

Step 13: Decluttering your Home

There's no limit to what you have to do to declutter your home; it actually depends on the amount of clutter you have lying around. Personally, it took me more than a week to make certain changes around my whole house. In some rooms, I had to simply move some things around while in others, I had to discard dozens of unnecessary belongings.

We've already been through decluttering our bedrooms, kitchen, pantry and closets in this book. The rest of the house isn't going to be very easy either. I'm just going to share a few decluttering tips that I followed in my journey that can help you make changes around the whole house.

Here they are:

- For the first step, take a trash bag in your hand and move through your house, going from room to room. In every room, you'll probably find something that should have been thrown away weeks ago, such as an empty bottle of shampoo in the bathroom, old receipts and bills, grocery lists, envelops and bank statements (be sure to tear them up first), pens that don't work, socks that have hole in them, expired makeup, old cell phone charger, and more. Depending on the type of hoarder that you are, it might take you more than one garbage bag and more than one trip to find things to throw away.

- Next, repeat the same step but this time, fill a bag with things to donate to Goodwill. This could be anything that you don't use but is in good shape. Examples? Barely used guest towels, baby clothes, old clothes that don't fit you anymore, old working phones and other gadgets, outdated kitchen appliances, dinner sets and Tupperware, comforters and baby blankets, old bedsheets and cushions, and everything else. If you donate them, these things will be available at an extremely affordable price to less fortunate people at thrift shops.

- If you have lots of items on display - on shelves, countertops, tabletops or cabinet tops, remove them all. Choose your favorite among them and put them back on display, and keep the rest aside. Your shelves and tabletops shouldn't be too cluttered with display items; there should ideally be only a few items on each. The ones you've removed can be donated or thrown away, or you can keep them in drawers and cupboards nearby. You can alternate between them to display on your walls and tabletops.

- Too many cushions on your couch can actually take up space. Only two to three cushions per couch is comfortable but exceeding that limit will leave most people no space to sit. Remove the excess if you have more cushions than what's comfortable.

- Remove everything that's not necessary in the long run, i.e. newspapers and magazines, take away menus from restaurants you don't plan on ordering from, wrapping paper kept for later, free samples from businesses, and more. These are the things we save thinking we'll need later, but never use.

- Children's rooms have the most items you can throw away to make room. Kids grow everything extremely fast, but their old possessions can help other less fortunate children. Their old clothes, blankets, shoes and school bags, completed coloring books and notebooks, broken crayons, old toys and story books – these might all be things you can donate or need to throw away.

- Technology has made a lot of physical possessions obsolete. Simply using a smartphone means you don't need to bother with a lot of items, namely DVDs, Audio CDs, calendars, torch lights and calculators, etc. If you don't have a working DVD player at home, do you need to treasure your old DVDs? Or your CDs? Do you need to hang a calendar on your walls, or keep a calculator in your drawer? Most of these things can be simply discarded.

- Most of the things that you haven't used for more than 12 months can be thrown away, except perhaps books, souvenirs, expensive couture outfits or photographs. So go through what's rarely unused in your house and you might be able to discard of a lot.

- All your paperwork can easily be digitized these days, which has limited the amount of files and folders we need to keep around. Everything that you don't need in a physical format can be shredded and discarded, only if the digital copy is safe in your computer.

- Anything that's easily available doesn't need to be saved for future use. Wrapping paper, phone chargers, magazines, cartons and packing boxes, Christmas decorations – all these items are available everywhere, so you don't have to bother saving them up.

There are hundreds of ways that you can start decluttering your home, many more than I can finish discussing in a single book. They will come automatically to you once you start; soon, you'll know exactly what should be saved and treasured around the house, and what needs to be discarded of immediately.

Step 14: Decluttering your Relationships

Now let's come to a completely different yet relevant topic: decluttering your relationships.

Not all relationships are equally important for us. While some people are the reason for our happiness, others can make us doubt ourselves. Almost of all us have some toxic relationships in our lives, which need to be decluttered as soon as possible. However, it's not so easy to simply discard people from our lives as we can do to old clothes and documents; it is still necessary, though.

Here's how to declutter toxic and harmful relationships from your life, which may take a minute or even months.

1. Distancing Yourself from People Who are Bad for you

Who are the topic people in your life? These are the friends, family members and colleagues who try to bring you bring, make you doubt yourself, regularly degrade or dismiss your opinions in front of others, has no regard for your emotions, and more. In short, you never feel good about yourself when you are with them or in their company. These kinds of toxic people are a part of everyone's life and they can severely damage our mental stability if we allow them to.

Toxicity can be in anyone: friends we have known from our childhood, close family members, colleagues and even our partners. Not every relationship stays the same forever; some may degrade to a harmful point over time. Even if this is someone you used to love and care about very much as one point of your life, it is very important to know the people who are bad for you.

So. How do you remove such people from your life?

Distancing yourself physically from them is the best idea. Try to avoid them in every way possible: stop going to gatherings where these people might be present, avoid their calls and decline their invitations or see them as infrequently as possible.

2. Avoid People Who Take Advantage

All through your life, you'll find people who'll only remember you when they need a favor or a handout. These are the people who take advantage of you. They don't really care about your wellbeing, but only seek to exploit you because you always try your best to help them.

It's a completely different factor when you are willing to help someone who is less fortunate than you, but another thing when you are being taken advantage of. These kinds of selfish people will make excuses when you ask them for a favor, but will readily ask you for help. It is extremely important that you distance yourself from these selfish and often ungrateful people.

To do this, it is crucial that you learn the subtle art of saying "no". Avoid their calls, decline their invitations and simply deny to help them any further. If you aren't used to saying "no" directly, make excuses. If they are smart, they'll get the hint and move on; if not, you'll just have to constantly avoid them for a long time. What's important is that you learn to discard the selfish people who are only in your life to take advantage of you.

3. Limit People who are Negative

Ideally, there shouldn't be any negative people in your life, but the situation cannot always be helped. Negative people can be really bad for your self-esteem, especially if they are always criticizing your decisions, undermining your achievements and draining your energy. These people are great at giving negative feedback and stopping others from achieving more.

The easiest way to deal with negative people is simply to stop listening to them. Just because someone is feeding you negative energy, it doesn't mean that you have to pay attention to them. It can be hard to avoid someone when you see them or interact with them regularly, like an unsupportive partner, a jealous sibling or a false friend. However, negative people need to go away from your life, even if it means that you stop talking to them, stop living with them or stop interacting with them in any way. What's important is that you declutter their words, thoughts and opinions from your life, even if you can't actually discard them from your life.

4. Avoid People who don't Believe in you

It is extremely important that you surround yourself with people who don't just believe in you, but also support and encourage you. For both men and women, being encourage to follow their dreams from loved ones is critical; without the support from the people around you, it is very difficult to do anything at all.

So, try and surround yourself with the people who believe in you, in your dreams and your capabilities. Whether you need encouragement in your professional, emotional, personal or spiritual life, make sure the people around you provide you with that. What about the people who doesn't believe in you? They simply have no place in your life.

5. Limit People You Don't Need in your Life

There's actually only a handful of people we need in our lives, a compilation of good friends, supportive family members, helpful neighbors and encouraging colleagues. Everyone else is redundant and unnecessary, such as the people we went to school with, the people we once lived beside, the colleagues from our previous jobs, fourth cousins twice removed, and distant members of our in-law families. Unless you have somehow grown closer to them over the years, you don't really need to interact with them regularly.

These are people you will perhaps meet once or twice every year, if not less. You don't really need to focus on them in your regular life. They don't need to be on your Social Media accounts or your phonebooks. Most importantly, they should be decluttered from your mind at other times when you are not in direct interaction with them.

Easier said than done, of course. It's not very easy to suddenly declutter all these people from your life, especially if you have known them intimately and for a long time. Here are some of the changes you can make.

- Avoid their phone calls. If they call repeatedly, pick up and make an excuse.
- Make excuses if they want to meet up.
- Make excuses if they want to come over. Be firm but diplomatic about it; you don't want to be insulting or disrespectful to anyone.
- Avoid gatherings or parties hosted by people you don't really want to get involved with.
- Talk only to a selected few people at social occasions.
- Host private celebrations with your family and a few loved ones instead of throwing a lavish affair.
- Minimize social gatherings with colleagues after work.
- Keep unwanted people out of your social media accounts.
- Filter what people see on your social media accounts.

What's important is to figure out the kind of people you should filter from your life, and follow through. You don't need to be a favorite among every single person that you know on this world; all you need to do is to focus on the people who are truly important to you and spend more time with them.

Step 15: Decluttering your Finances

Finally, on to one of the most important topic in this book: decluttering your finances.

You might think it difficult to find any similarities between decluttering your home and your finances, but they are closely related. There's absolutely no use in cleaning your home and discarding of everything unnecessary when your finances are a mess. Perhaps this is the first cleaning up you should start with, depending on your situation; or, this could be the perfect way to finish your decluttering journey.

For most of us, our financial situation can get complicated if we are not complicated. With one (or two) income sources and thousands of expenditures, it is easy for anyone to get confused once in a while. Your finances need proper management, even when your expenses are pretty straightforward.

My finances were in a huge mess when I first started. With two incomes, multiple bank accounts and credit cards, hundreds of cash and non-cash transactions, our family's finances used to confuse me whenever I sat down with it. Most importantly, there were a number of unnecessary and extravagant expenses that were cutting down on our incomes. It was important for us to decide as a family the exact expenses we want to discard from our home.

Too many debts, too many credit cards, too many bank accounts, too many expenditures. We had to make a sense of things, and it was impossible to do so without decluttering our finances the proper way.

At the end, here's what we did:

- We combined our bank accounts and brought them down to three. One account where my income came in and one in which my partner's income came in, and a joint account we both used for household expenses. Every month, we'd transfer a fixed amount of money to our joint account that is to be used for all the household expenditure.

-We each got two credit/debit cards, as opposed to the half a dozen cards we used previously. One was for our household expenditures and the other for our personal expenditures or emergencies.

-Every single debt we had was brought under one bank account where we both paid a particular amount of money every day. We had around 5 to 6 loans and debts in total, both to banks and individuals. We paid up the small debts and bought everything else under one bank account, making payment every month easier.

-We actually made money from selling all the expensive things around the house we didn't need or use, although at a rate lower than the cost price. This included our old DVD collection, certain paintings, vintage clothes and unworn shoes, couture bags and other expensive things. This reduced the clutter in our house and helped us make some extra cash. We used this cash to pay away a few debts.

-We cancelled our random and spontaneous weekend getaways and mini-holidays, and instead, started saving for one lavish vacation every year. This simplified the expenses as a certain amount of money started going into our vacation fund every month.

-We reduced the number of subscriptions to different magazines, and music and streaming networks. Instead, we decided on one for a few months and changed the options every few months.

-We automated certain payments so that they were already paid by the time we started spending for our household expenses, i.e. mortgage, utility bill, school fees.

-We made a list of everything we need for the house every month, and tried to follow it strictly.

-We used a single credit card/bank account to pay all the bills and mandatory expenses, so it is easier to know what amount of money was used in which purpose.

-We started to save all of our receipts and bill, but instead of cluttering up our drawers, we stored them digitally.

These are only some of the steps we took to stop being a hostage of our financial situation and to be honest, it helped us a lot. We could finally, after years of struggling, make sense of our money. We knew exactly what we were spending and where our money was going, and we were successful in stopping wasteful expenditures.

Conclusion

Decluttering doesn't mean to simply go through your belongings and throw away empty bottles and expired food. It is much bigger than that. When you declutter your life, you can find out exactly how little you need to live a good life and how something that has been gathering dust in your closet can bring comfort to someone else. Decluttering makes you responsible, so that you can be mindful of your purchases in the future.

Decluttering shouldn't just be limited to your closet or your pantry, but to every part of your life. The people who don't bring you joy, the responsibilities that feel like obligations, the relationships that are dragging you down, the friends who clearly don't want to see you succeed – these are the aspects of your life that also need to be decluttered.

In this book, I have tried to discuss every single way that you can make your life simple and stress-free. From throwing away everything that clutters up your room to every person who makes your life complicated, there is a way to let go of everything and everyone. All you have to do is to recognize the aspects of your life that needs decluttering and organizing, and get to work.

Hopefully, you have gotten some idea about how to start decluttering your life from this book. These were mostly steps and tricks I have followed in my personal decluttering journey, as well as research based on other people's experiences. If you had liked even some of them, I would consider my book to be a success.

Thank you for reading!

Jennifer N. Smith

Jennifer N. Smith

9 798647 815514